VEGETARIAN DIET COOKBOOK

THE ESSENTIAL GUIDE TO VEGETARIAN DIETING

HEATHER PEAKE

Table of Contents

CHAPTER ONE

vegetarian diet

According to a new study, the vegetarian diet has the same weight-loss potential as the Mediterranean diet. Furthermore, the "bad" LDL cholesterol was reduced more effectively on the vegetarian diet. 1 When it comes to getting healthy, there are so many options out there that it can be overwhelming. However, vegetarianism is becoming more and more popular as a way to boost energy, fitness, and overall health.

It's easier than ever to eat a plant-based diet and call yourself a "veggie" nowadays. Starting with plant-based meat substitutes, which have grown in popularity due to heightened public awareness in the United States, there are a growing number of delicious recipes and establishments that cater specifically to vegetarians and vegans. If you're curious about how it can aid in weight loss and what the best practices are, read on! Here's a quick download from the experts on the vegetarian diet.

The term "vegetarian diet" is used to describe a diet that excludes animal products.

It isn't nearly as restrictive as other plant-based diets, and many vegetarians still eat eggs and dairy products, despite the fact that meat consumption is forbidden. Individuals who use this method of eating do so for a variety of reasons, including those related to their health, religion or environment, or even their own cultural heritage. There are a number of health considerations to take into account before making any major changes in your diet.

Vegetarianism is most commonly referred to as "Lacto-Ovo," a type of vegetarianism that does not include animal products but does allow for dairy and eggs, says Lon Ben-Asher. As well as "Ovo," which allows eggs, and "vegan," which bans all meat and animal products, the nutritionist cites these two other popular vegetarian diets. Next, we'll discuss the most common type of vegetarianism, which allows for eggs, dairy, and other animal by-products while ignoring meat.

Why you may be unable to shed the pounds you've put on.

Those who follow a diet high in fat, moderate in protein, and low in starch and carbs do better at losing weight than those who follow a more traditional diet.

For the most part, people on low-carb diets fared better than those on low-fat diets when it came to sustaining long-term weight loss. Because they consumed fewer carbohydrates, people on high-fat diets performed better than those on low-fat diets.

Many studies have shown that when you eat a diet high in protein and fat, your lean body mass increases, while your fat mass decreases.

For those who are unable to shed the pounds on a vegetarian diet, here are some possible explanations.

You're overindulging in food calorically.

When eaten in large quantities, legumes, nuts, and seeds, which are all sources of protein, are high in calories.

Eating more of these foods than meat is necessary for a vegetarian to meet their protein requirements," says Zumpano. When it comes to protein, a 4-ounce piece of lean meat provides about 200 calories and 28 grams of protein. Cooked beans provide close to 400 calories to get the same amount of protein as that found in two cups of cooked beans."

Similarly, a 1-ounce serving of nuts provides 200 calories and the same amount of protein as a 1-ounce piece of lean meat, but the meat only has 55 calories.

Beans are a good source of protein and carbohydrate, so treat them as such when preparing a meal. Refrain from adding another carb, like potatoes, pasta or rice," Zumpano advises. As a result, you should eat more beans in order to meet your protein requirements."

If you're looking for a low-carb source of protein like tofu, seitan, tempeh, or a dairy product like Greek yogurt or cottage cheese, you can also opt for egg whites or egg white substitutes.

You're consuming far too many refined carbs.

Vegetarians can, in fact, consume carbs. However, overconsumption of refined carbohydrates is a common blunder. Pizza, pasta, and bread are all on the menu.

They are low in fiber and leave you with an unsatisfying feeling of fullness after eating. As a result, you're more likely to overindulge.

You should instead eat a diet rich in sweet potatoes and butternut squash as well as oatmeal and beans and lentils. Because they don't cause your blood sugar to spike as quickly, these fiber-rich complex carbohydrate options are preferable.

CHAPTER TWO

As long as you keep your portion sizes in check and always include a protein source and plenty of vegetables when you eat pizza or pasta, it's fine to indulge once in a while," says Zumpano. Pasta primavera with various vegetables and chickpeas or lentils for protein, for example." Make a veggie pizza with fresh mozzarella and serve it with a salad."

Too many high-calorie foods are being consumed.

The natural fat content of foods like nuts, butters, seeds, avocados and coconut may help you feel full and satisfied while on a vegetarian diet. Foods like these are nutritious and filling. But even a small amount goes a long way, so it's easy to overeat.

Keep a food and drink diary to track your intake and identify any foods that are packing on the pounds and preventing you from slimming down, advises Zumpano. Consider using a calorie-tracking app or a notebook to keep track of what you eat. "

You're eating highly processed foods

Eliminating meat from your diet increases your intake of processed foods.

However, despite the fact that many of these products are labeled "vegetarian," they contain a wide range of unhealthy ingredients such as added sugar and sodium as well as artificial preservatives and flavorings.

Zumpano gushes, "These foods are both convenient and delicious. It's important to keep track of your caloric intake to ensure that you don't overeat on these foods.

Nutritional advantages of vegetarianism

The health benefits of eating more plant-based foods even if you occasionally eat meat outweigh the drawbacks. People who follow a plant-based diet are less likely to suffer from heart disease, certain cancers, or diabetes. In addition, those who adhere to plant-based diets tend to be more successful in their weight loss efforts. Why is this so? Fruits, vegetables, nuts, seeds, whole grains, and legumes are all good sources of fiber, which is the bulk of the diet. This nutrient helps us feel fuller for longer, which means we eat fewer calories in the long run. Discover the health benefits of consuming more fiber by reading this article.

When You're Eating a Plant-Based Diet

- Lentils and beans

Nuts and seed butters (including chia and flax)

Grains of all kinds (quinoa, bulgur, freekeh, whole-wheat, oats, brown rice and more)

Soybean (tofu, edamame, tempeh)

- Fruits

- Vegetables

• Dairy is an important source of protein (yogurt, kefir, cheese, milk)

• Eggs

Omega-3 fatty acids (such as olives, olive oil, avocado)

A Vegetarian's Guide to Weight Loss

According to Food Effect author and nutritionist "[One study of obese individuals found] that most men and women lose weight when they switch to eating plant-based protein instead of red meat and animal protein." The vegetarian diet is beneficial for weight loss. She also cited studies showing that people were more likely to become overweight or obese if they consumed more animal protein and saturated fats.

weight loss is all about creating a calorie deficit. What is his word of wisdom? Pay attention to the calorie content. To help you feel fuller longer, choose foods that are low in calories but high in water and dietary fiber. This will fill up your stomach and keep you satisfied for longer. Fruits, vegetables, whole grains, and legumes are examples of minimally processed foods. Keep in mind, though, that you don't want to go too low on calories. There must be no severe restrictions in order to achieve long-term health and weight loss.

As a side note, if you're lactose intolerant, you may not be able to get enough protein from your diet, which is essential for a well-balanced diet. It's possible, though. If you're a vegetarian, Braude has some good advice on how to get enough protein into your diet.

Even the strongest primate, the gorilla, gets all the protein and iron it needs by eating nothing but fruit, vegetables and leaves. "This should give you some idea of how much protein and iron the gorilla gets by not eating animal protein," she says. According to her, "a human vegetarian diet is likely to be more varied, with plenty of plant-based protein (nuts, nut butter, legumes and so on) so you definitely have nothing to worry about."

CHAPTER THREE

What Vegetarian Foods Help You Lose Weight Faster than Other Foods?

vegetarians should eat a lot of unrefined carbohydrates and grains like oatmeal, quinoa, buckwheat and farro. They should also consume a lot of vegetables and fruits like potatoes and yams. After giving up meat, Braude says it's important to make sure you're getting enough protein in your diet. In order to ensure that you're getting enough protein, the author and nutritionist created a helpful table that you can use to figure out how much meat substitutes to eat each day:

As many as 75 grams of prepared lentils (18g protein)

- 75 grams of split peas, cooked (16g protein)

- 2 hens' eggs (12g protein)

250 g plain Greek yogurt, 0% fat (23g protein)

- 100 grams of raw oats (7g protein)

- 1 yam or other tuber (4g protein)

In addition to 40g of chia seeds (12g protein)

- 25g of whey protein (20–25g protein)

sunflower seeds, 4 tbsp (8g protein)

Which Vegetarian Foods Should You AVOID When Trying to Lose Weight?

There are numerous health benefits to reducing your meat consumption, but not all plant-based foods are equal. It's best to avoid eating large quantities of "packaged and highly-processed foods," such as potato chips, pretzels, dried cereals, bread, and crackers, according to Ben-Asher. Eating whole foods rather than restricting yourself to one or more food groups or types is healthier (and simpler) in the long run.

Some of the calorie counting is already done for you if you

follow a vegetarian diet. Animal protein, especially meat, contains a lot of saturated fat, so cutting it out of your diet will help you lose weight, says Braude. According to her, some cuts of poultry, such as dark chicken with the skin on, are "extremely high in fat and therefore calories" despite their "healthy" label.

How to Prepare a Week's Worth of Meals in Advance:

The Lemon-Roasted Vegetable Hummus Bowls can be meal prepped the day before and taken to work with you in to-go containers.

To enjoy throughout the week, prepare a batch of the Baked Banana-Nut Oatmeal Cups in advance. To preserve freshness, store in airtight meal-prep containers.

Snack on the Peanut-Butter Energy Balls this week for a tasty afternoon pick-me-up. It can be stored in an airtight container in the refrigerator for up to 5 days, or in the freezer for up to 3 months.

Make three hard-boiled eggs for the week's worth of snacks.

The first day of school

a hearty and filling start to (310 calories)

- 1 1/2 cups water and 3/4 cup oats cooked together

- One-third cup of raspberry

Add raspberries and a pinch of cinnamon to the oatmeal.

Snack in the Morning (95 calories)

• 1 medium-sized apple

To eat (345 calories)

Whole Wheat Veggie Wrap • 1 serving

Snack of the Day for the Afternoon (80 calories)

At least half a cup of nonfat Greek yogurt

Sliced strawberries, about one-fourth cup

Afternoon meal (394 calories)

Mushroom-Quinoa Veggie Burgers with a Special Sauce: 1 serving

1,224 calories, 45 grams of protein, 173 grams of carbohydrates, 33 grams of fiber, 43 grams of fat, 1,269 milligrams of sodium.

The second day.

a hearty and filling start to (211 calories)

Oatmeal Cups Baked Banana-Nut

- 1 clementine per person

Snack in the Morning (116 calories)

- 1/4 cup of raspberries.

Three-quarters of a cup of nonfat Greek yogurt

To eat (360 calories)

The Lemon-Roasted Vegetable Hummus Bowls serve one person

Snack of the Day for the Afternoon (174 calories)

Energy Balls Made with Peanut Butter

Afternoon meal (422 calories)

Squash and Black Bean Tostadas with Butternut Squash

1,214 calories, 51 grams of protein, 163 grams of carbohydrates, 32 grams of fiber, 47 grams of fat, and 1,317 milligrams of sodium make up the daily totals.

CHAPTER FOUR

The third day.

a hearty and filling start to (271 calories)

Oatmeal Cups Baked Banana-Nut

- 1 medium-sized apple

Snack in the Morning (78 calories)

With a pinch of salt and pepper, you can season a hard-boiled egg

To eat (360 calories)

The Lemon-Roasted Vegetable Hummus Bowls serve one person

Snack of the Day for the Afternoon (32 calories)

1/4 cup of red currants

Afternoon meal (380 calories)

2 Tbsp. shredded Parmesan cheese on top of 1 serving One-Pot Tomato Bail Pasta.

In the Evening (174 calories)

Energy Balls Made with Peanut Butter

1,208 calories, 55 grams of protein, 160 grams of carbohydrates, 32 grams of fiber, 45 grams of fat, 1,478 milligrams of sodium per day.

After the fourth day,

a hearty and filling start to (271 calories)

Oatmeal Cups Baked Banana-Nut

- 1 medium-sized apple

Snack in the Morning (78 calories)

With a pinch of salt and pepper, you can season a hard-boiled egg

To eat (360 calories)

The Lemon-Roasted Vegetable Hummus Bowls serve one person

Snack of the Day for the Afternoon (35 calories)

- 1 clementine per person

Afternoon meal (405 calories)

- 2 Tbsp. shredded Cheddar cheese and 1 Tbsp. sour cream on top of 1 serving of Stuffed Potatoes with Salsa and Beans

In the Evening (174 calories)

Energy Balls Made with Peanut Butter

A daily intake of 1,215 calories, 49 grams of protein, 162 grams of carbohydrates, 32 grams of fiber, 46 grams of fat, and 1,349 milligrams of sodium is considered healthy for most people.

The fifth day has come.

a hearty and filling start to (306 calories)

• 1 serving of Avocado-Egg Toast. •

• 1 clementine per person

Snack in the Morning (32 calories)

1/4 cup of red currants

To eat (360 calories)

The Lemon-Roasted Vegetable Hummus Bowls serve one person

Snack of the Day for the Afternoon (95 calories)

• 1 medium-sized apple

Afternoon meal (428 calories)

Vegetarian Tikka Masala

• 3/4 of a cup of brown rice that has been cooked

The daily totals include 1,221 calories, 47 g protein, 155 g carbohydrates, 35 g fiber, 53 g fat, 1,203 mg sodium.

The sixth day of the challenge.

a hearty and filling start to (310 calories)

- 1 1/2 cups water and 3/4 cup oats cooked together

- One-third cup of raspberry

Add raspberries and a pinch of cinnamon to the oatmeal.

Snack of the Day for the Afternoon (95 calories)

- 1 medium-sized apple

To eat (345 calories)

Whole Wheat Veggie Wrap • 1 serving

Snack of the Day for the Afternoon (174 calories)

Energy Balls Made with Peanut Butter

Afternoon meal (360 calories)

• 1 serving of vegan tacos without meat

There are 1,225 calories in a day in this diet. There are 44 grams of protein, 165 grams of carbohydrate, 35 grams of fiber, and 49 grams of fat.

The seventh day has come.

a hearty and filling start to (322 calories)

oatmeal cooked with half a cup of water and skim milk, half a cup of water

- Diced up half a medium apple

Chopped walnuts, about a tablespoonful

Snack in the Morning (95 calories)

• 1 medium-sized apple

To eat (345 calories)

Whole Wheat Veggie Wrap • 1 serving

Snack of the Day for the Afternoon (78 calories)

With a pinch of salt and pepper, you can season a hard-boiled egg

Afternoon meal (401 calories)

Curry Chickpea Stew, 1 serving

Dietary Values Per Day (Calories), Protein (67 G), Carbohydrates (138 G), Fiber (31 G), Fat (46 G), Sodium (1,625 mg).

The Ending Thoughts

Consult a nutritionist or doctor before making any major changes to your diet, especially if you plan to drastically reduce your meat consumption. Veganism is a viable option for some people, but it's important to check in with yourself frequently to ensure that going "veggie" is the right choice for you in terms of nutrition.

Reduce your intake of animal products and byproducts while increasing your intake of whole foods (vegetables, whole grains, and fruits) and a variety of plant-based protein sources at the same time. If weight loss is your ultimate goal, keep in mind that the number on the scale is not always the best indicator of health. There are numerous health benefits and advantages to a vegetarian diet that have nothing to do with weight loss, weight gain, or maintenance.

THE END